CPR Made Simple
Full Master Edition
By Munashe Davies Gumbo

Nurse, BLS/ CPR Instructor, Founder – OM Good Samaritan
First Edition – 2025

© 2025 Munashe Gumbo | All Rights Reserved
www.goodsamaritanca.com

Dedication

Dedicated to every bystander, caregiver, and healthcare worker who has ever stepped forward to save a life. Every heartbeat you restored kept someone else's story alive.

Preface – Why I Wrote This Book

Cardiac arrest is one of the leading causes of death worldwide, yet many lives can be saved each year through prompt and effective cardiopulmonary resuscitation (CPR).

Too often, people hesitate—because of fear, uncertainty, or the assumption that "someone else knows better." I have seen hesitation cost precious seconds and sometimes a life. **Every minute lost without oxygenated blood supply to the brain results in about 10% of the brain dying reducing chances of survival.** I have also seen the opposite: a moment of courage that turns panic into purpose and hopelessness into a heartbeat.

As a nurse and CPR instructor, I have stood in both worlds—the quiet before a code blue and the coordinated rush that brings someone back. I wrote this book to bridge that gap for everyone: students, parents, caregivers, and any person who might be present when a life hangs in the balance.

This book does not replace formal certification. Rather, it gives you the knowledge and confidence to recognize an emergency, respond appropriately, and understand **why** immediate action matters. You don't need to be a doctor or nurse to save a life—you need willingness to learn, remember, and act.

Every story and real-life example here grows from a simple truth: an ordinary person, with the right knowledge and courage, can do something extraordinary.

I hope these pages empower you to be that person—the one who steps forward when every second counts.

CHAPTER INDEX

Chapter 1 – Understanding Basic Life Support / CPR

Chapter 2 – What Is CPR and Why It Matters

Chapter 3 – The Chain of Survival

Chapter 4 – When to Start and Stop CPR

Chapter 5 – Step-by-Step Guide to CPR

Chapter 6 – AED Basics and How to Use One

Chapter 7 – Understanding Code Status (Full Code vs DNR)

Chapter 8 – Common Mistakes and Myths About CPR

Chapter 9 – Emotional and Ethical Aspects of Resuscitation

Chapter 10 – Choking (Adults, Infants, Pregnant & LifeVac)

Chapter 11 – Living Through CPR: Realities, Gratitude & Courage

Chapter 1 – Understanding Basic Life Support / CPR

What CPR Does
Cardiopulmonary resuscitation (CPR) is a lifesaving technique that keeps oxygen-rich blood flowing to the brain and vital organs until the heart's normal rhythm can be restored. Since its adoption in the 1960s, CPR has helped save millions of lives.

CPR combines two critical actions:
- **Chest compressions** to manually pump blood through the body.
- **Rescue breaths** to deliver oxygen to the lungs (added when trained and equipped).

What the words mean
- **Cardio** = heart
- **Pulmonary** = lungs
- **Resuscitation** = to revive

The heart is an electrical pump. During cardiac arrest, its electrical signals fail, and the heart can't pump effectively. Chest compressions become a temporary engine for circulation.

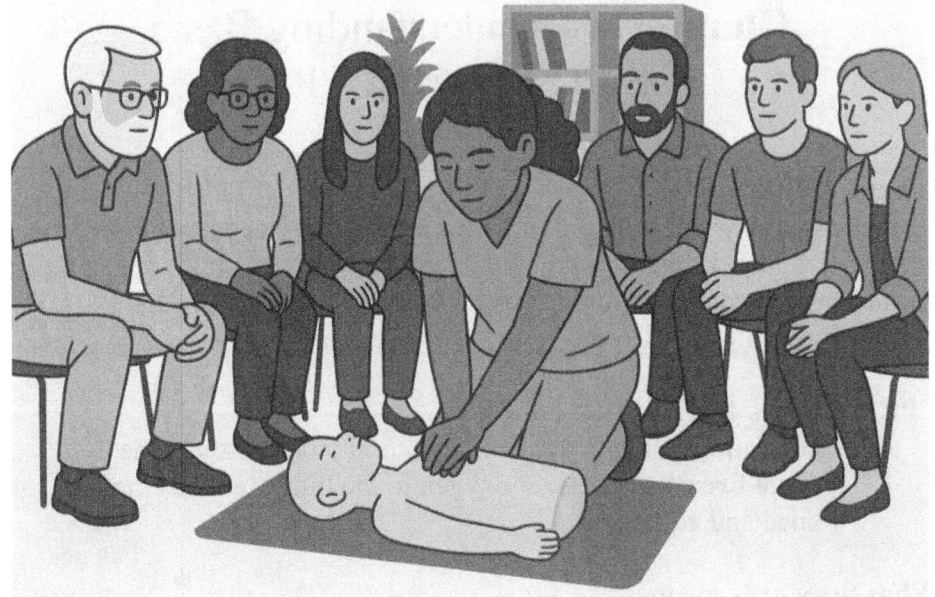

Figure 1

Heart Attack vs. Cardiac Arrest

These terms are often confused:
- **Heart Attack (Myocardial Infarction):** A blockage interrupts blood flow to part of the heart muscle. The person is usually awake and breathing.
- **Cardiac Arrest:** The heart's electrical system malfunctions; the person becomes unresponsive and stops breathing normally.

A heart attack can lead to cardiac arrest, but not always. When arrest occurs, act immediately. Survival falls sharply with each minute without CPR and defibrillation. Begin CPR right away.

Some individuals choose **DNR (Do Not Resuscitate)** orders because they do not wish to be revived, often due to expected poor quality of life after prolonged oxygen loss. If a valid DNR is unavailable, treat it as **Full Code**.

CAB vs. ABC — The Modern Sequence

Older teaching emphasized **A-B-C** (Airway, Breathing, Circulation). Current guidelines prioritize **C-A-B** (Circulation, Airway, Breathing).

Why the change?
Delays in compressions reduce blood flow to the brain and heart. Start compressions first. If fluid or vomit is present, roll the person briefly to the side (≤10 seconds) to clear the mouth, then resume compressions immediately.

Hesitation Barriers & Safety

Modesty and the "Breast Factor"
Out-of-hospital survival is lower for women in part due to hesitation about exposing the chest. Good-faith rescuers are generally protected by Good Samaritan laws. Removing or cutting clothing to place hands correctly and apply AED pads is appropriate and time critical. If removing clothing would cause delay, start compressions over clothing while preparing to expose the chest safely.

Scene and Surface Check

Before compressions, perform a rapid visual check: hazards (wires, traffic, fluids), objects under clothing (patches, needles, lodged objects). Expose the chest as soon as feasible for accurate hand placement and AED pad placement.

In another incident, a rescuer pressed down on a victim lying in a pool of blood — unaware this person had been stabbed from the back, and a knife was lodged in the chest. His hands pressed right into the knife, and he became the second victim.

Consider some drug overdose cases — you may encounter needles under clothing or hidden objects. Expose the chest safely whenever possible.

Quick Reference: Adult CPR Priorities

1. **Check safety** of the scene.
2. **Check responsiveness**: tap and shout.

3. **Call for help / activate EMS** (use speakerphone).
4. **Check breathing** and, if trained, **check pulse** for 5–10 seconds.
5. **Start compressions** in the center of the chest (lower half of the sternum).
6. **Rate** 100–120/min; **depth** at least 2 in (5 cm); allow **full recoil**.
7. **Minimize interruptions**; apply **AED** as soon as available.

Why Chest Recoil Matters

After you press hard and fast on the chest, you must let it fully spring back up before the next push. That "rise" is the chest recoil- it's how the heart refills with blood so your next compression can actually push blood out again. If you don't let it rise, the heart can't refill- it's like trying to pump a flat sponge without letting it expand.

Think of the heart like a pump handle: pushing down ejects blood; letting the chest fully rise refills the heart. Incomplete recoil starves the next compression.

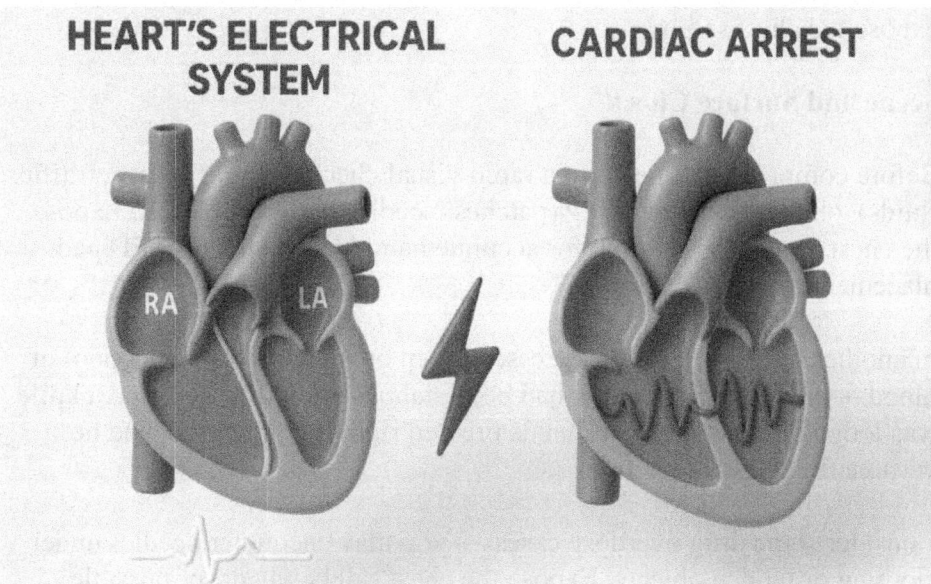

Figure 2: Basic Illustration of Heart's Electrical System and Cardiac Arrest

Chapter 2 – What CPR Is and Why It Matters

When a person's heart stops, oxygen stops reaching the brain and other vital organs. CPR keeps blood flowing long enough for advanced care to arrive — it is a bridge between collapse and recovery.

Hands-Only CPR (for untrained rescuers)

If you have not been formally trained or don't have a barrier device:

Do:
Continuous chest compressions in the center of the chest at 100-120 per minute, at least 2 inches (5cm) deep, with full chest recoil.

Don't:
Pause for rescue breaths. Early, uninterrupted compressions keep blood moving, and most adults have residual oxygen for the first few minutes.

Conventional CPR (for trained rescuers)

If trained and equipped with a barrier device:

- **Cycle: 30 Compressions: 2 Breaths** (about 1 second per breath, just enough for visible chest rise)
- **Minimize interruptions:** Resume compressions immediately after each breath and after any AED analysis or shock.

Key point: Compressions are the priority. Every pause lowers coronary (heart) and cerebral (brain) perfusion.

Why It Matters

CPR gives the body a *fighting chance* until medical help arrives. It keeps the brain alive.

- **Protects the brain.** Brain injury begins within minutes of untreated cardiac arrest. High-quality compressions slow that clock.
- **Buys time for defibrillation.** Most adult out of hospital arrests are due to shockable rhythms like ventricular fibrillation (VF), which

is a life-threatening heart rhythm in which the ventricles quiver chaotically instead of contracting in a coordinated way. CPR keeps organs perfused, so a shock has better chances to work.
- **Transforms bystanders into lifesavers.** Immediate action by the first person on scene is often the difference between recovery and irreversible damage.

When to Add Breaths
- **Adults:** Hands-only is acceptable if untrained. If trained and with a barrier device, **use 30:2**
- **Children and infants:** Cardiac arrest is more often breathing-related; **breaths are important.** If alone and untrained, perform compressions, if trained, **use 30:2 (single rescuer)** or **15:2 (two or more rescuers).**

Practical Tips for Quality Compressions

- Hard, flat surface when possible
- Shoulders staked directly over hands; elbows locked.
- Count out loud at a rate of 100-120 compressions per minute.
- Rotate compressors every 2 minutes if help is available to prevent fatigue.
- Avoid leaning on the chest- full recoil matters

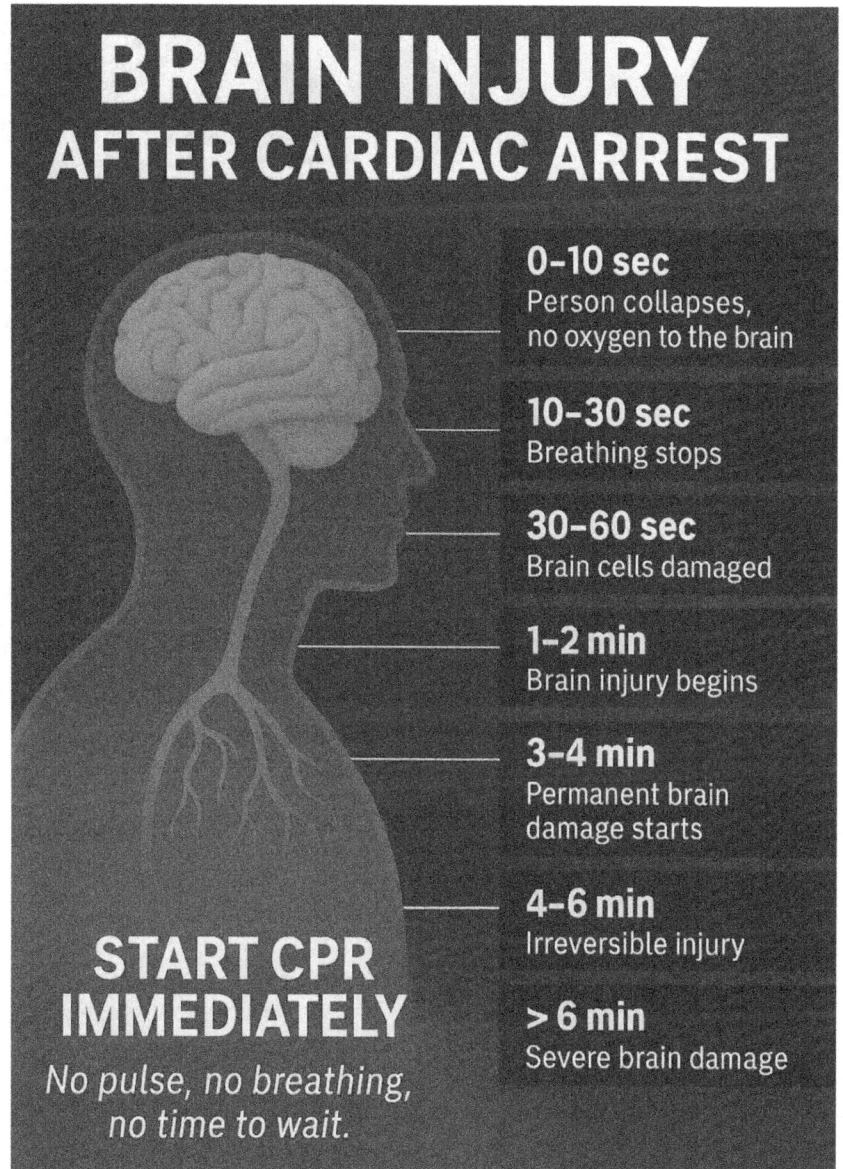

Figure 3- Brain cells begin to die within minutes of cardiac arrest. Starting CPR immediately keeps oxygen flowing and protects the brain until a normal heartbeat returns.

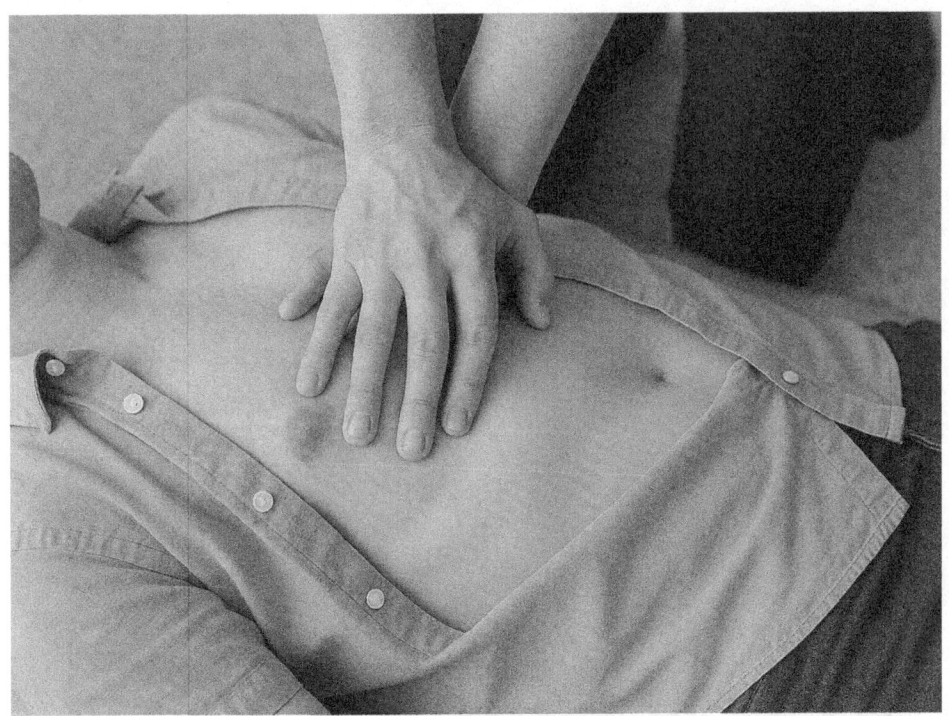

Figure 4 – Correct Hand Placement for Adult Chest Compressions

Chapter 3 – The Chain of Survival

The Five (Now Six) Links in the Chain of Survival

1. **Prevention and Preparedness**

Recognize high-risk individuals and environments.
Promote heart-healthy habits, early medical intervention, and public access to defibrillators (AEDs).
Prevention is the first, often overlooked, step that reduces the need for CPR altogether.

2. **Early Recognition & Call for Help**

- Recognize cardiac arrest and activate the emergency response system immediately.
- Call 911 (or your emergency local number).
- Put your phone on speaker.
- Follow the dispatcher's instructions step-by-step.
- If possible, send someone to retrieve an AED.

3. **Early CPR**

Start compressions immediately to keep blood flowing to the brain and heart.
- High-quality compressions mean:
- Rate: 100–120/min
- Depth: at least 2 inches (5 cm) for adults
- Full recoil between compressions
- Minimal interruptions

4. **Early Defibrillation**

Use an Automated External Defibrillator (AED) as soon as it becomes available.

Defibrillation restores the heart's normal rhythm in shockable cases (ventricular fibrillation or pulseless ventricular tachycardia).
Each minute without defibrillation decreases survival by roughly 7–10%.

5. **Advanced Life Support (ALS)**

Once emergency responders arrive, they provide advanced airway management, medications, and cardiac monitoring to restore spontaneous circulation.

Post–Cardiac Arrest Care

After return of spontaneous circulation (ROSC), which in simple terms is the return of pulse. Focus shifts to protecting the brain and heart.

Intensive care includes:
- Maintaining oxygenation and blood pressure
- Managing temperature (targeted temperature management)
- Treating underlying causes

If one link fails, the chain weakens.

The Process – Step-by-Step Response Let's imagine you encounter an unresponsive person:

a) Check the scene for safety.
Ensure there are no dangers — live wires, vehicles, bodily fluids, or other hazards.

b) Check responsiveness.
Tap the shoulders firmly and shout, "Are you OK? Are you OK?"

Never shake the person — if they've had a fall or possible spinal injury, shaking may worsen it.

c) Check for breathing and a pulse (if trained).

- **Adults:** Use the carotid pulse — two fingers on the trachea, slide into the groove beside the windpipe. Check for 5–10 seconds while observing chest movement.
- **Infants:** Use the brachial pulse on the inside of the upper arm.

If no normal breathing and no pulse, or if you're unsure — treat as **cardiac arrest** and start CPR immediately.

d) Activate emergency response.

Call 911 (or your local number). If alone, put your phone on speaker and follow dispatcher instructions step-by-step.

e) Start CPR.
Begin compressions in the center of the chest. If trained, add breaths at a 30: 2 ratio. If an AED is present, turn it on immediately and follow its prompts.

f) Continue CPR.
Don't stop until one of the following happens: the person starts breathing normally, paramedics take over, or you are physically unable to continue.

g) Direct others clearly.

If you're leading the scene, give specific commands:
- "John, call 911."
- "Mary, start compressions."
- "You in the blue shirt, bring the AED."
- Avoid vague phrases like "Someone call 911" — that causes the **bystander effect**, where everyone assumes someone else has already acted.

Key Concept: Every second Counts
- Early Recognition- Early Activation
- Early Compressions- Maintained Circulation

- Early defibrillation- Restored Rhythm

Remember:
When these links happen seamlessly, survival rates rise dramatically. Early action saves lives. Courage comes before confidence. Every compression buys time for the heart and brain.

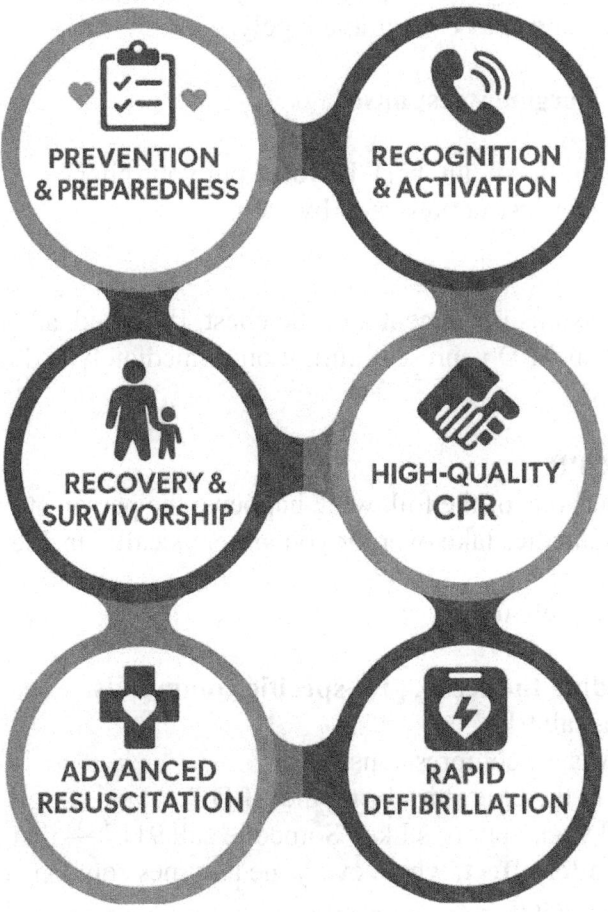

Figure 5 – Chain of Survival Diagram

Chapter 4 – When to Start and Stop CPR

If a person collapses, is **unresponsive**, and **not breathing normally**, **start CPR immediately**. If you're trained, check a pulse for **no more than 5–10 seconds** while assessing breathing. If there's **no definite pulse** or you're **unsure—begin compressions now**.

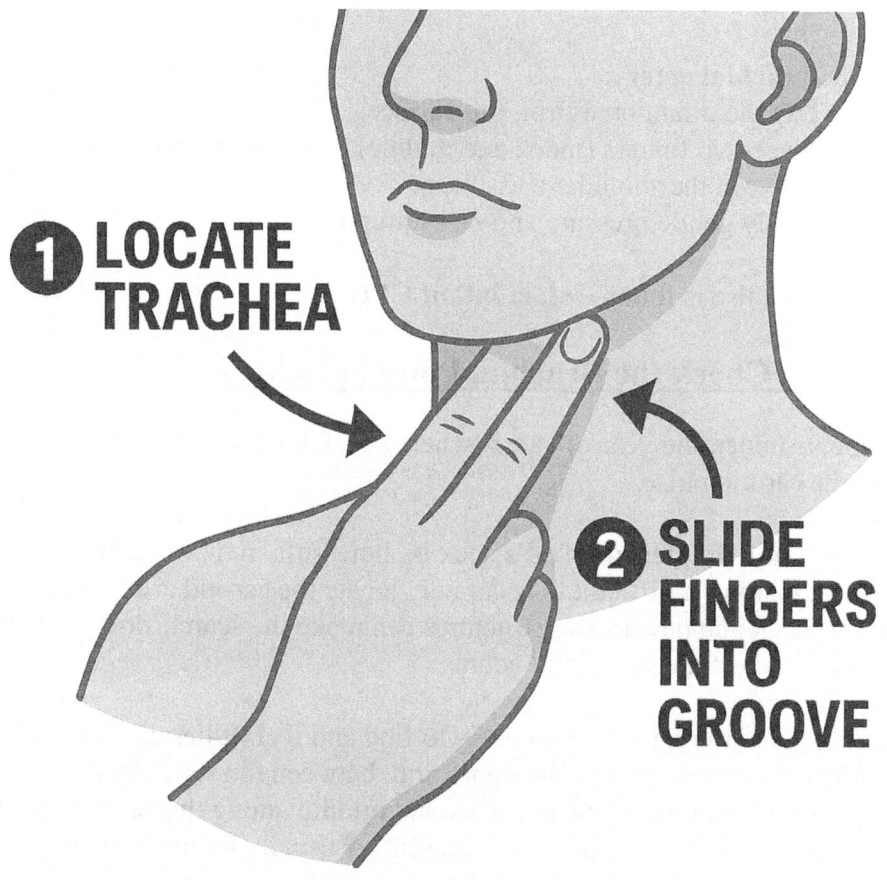

Figure 6- Carotid Pulse

Quick Start: Adult & Child (≥1 year)

Pulse check (for trained rescuers):
Use the carotid artery.

1. Place two fingers on the trachea (front of the neck).
2. Slide into the groove beside the windpipe.
3. Feel for a pulse **for no more than 10 seconds.**

If no pulse is felt—or un-sure—**start chest compressions immediately.**

Tip: For children, the **carotid or femoral pulse** is acceptable. If you're not confident finding either, skip the pulse check and **start compressions.**

Infants (Birth–1 year)

Use the **brachial artery.**
1. Lay the infant on a firm, flat surface.
2. Place two fingers (index and middle) on the inner upper arm, between the shoulder and elbow.
3. Apply gentle pressure and feel for up to 10 seconds.

If no clear pulse is found—**start infant CPR.**

Why We Check the Brachial Pulse in Infants

In infants under one year of age, rescuers check the brachial pulse rather than the carotid pulse.

The reason is simple: an infant's neck is short, soft, and not yet well-defined, making it difficult to accurately locate the carotid artery. Their chubby neck and developing structures can make the search slow — and in cardiac arrest, every second counts.

The brachial artery, however, is easy to find and feel. It lies close to the surface on the inner part of the upper arm, between the shoulder and elbow. By placing two fingers (index and middle) along this area, rescuers can quickly determine if a pulse is present — usually within 5 to 10 seconds.

Pro Tip
- Avoid using your thumb — it has its own pulse and can confuse you.
- Apply gentle pressure; pressing too hard can collapse the small artery.

- Check one arm only — never both.

CHECK BRACHIAL PULSE

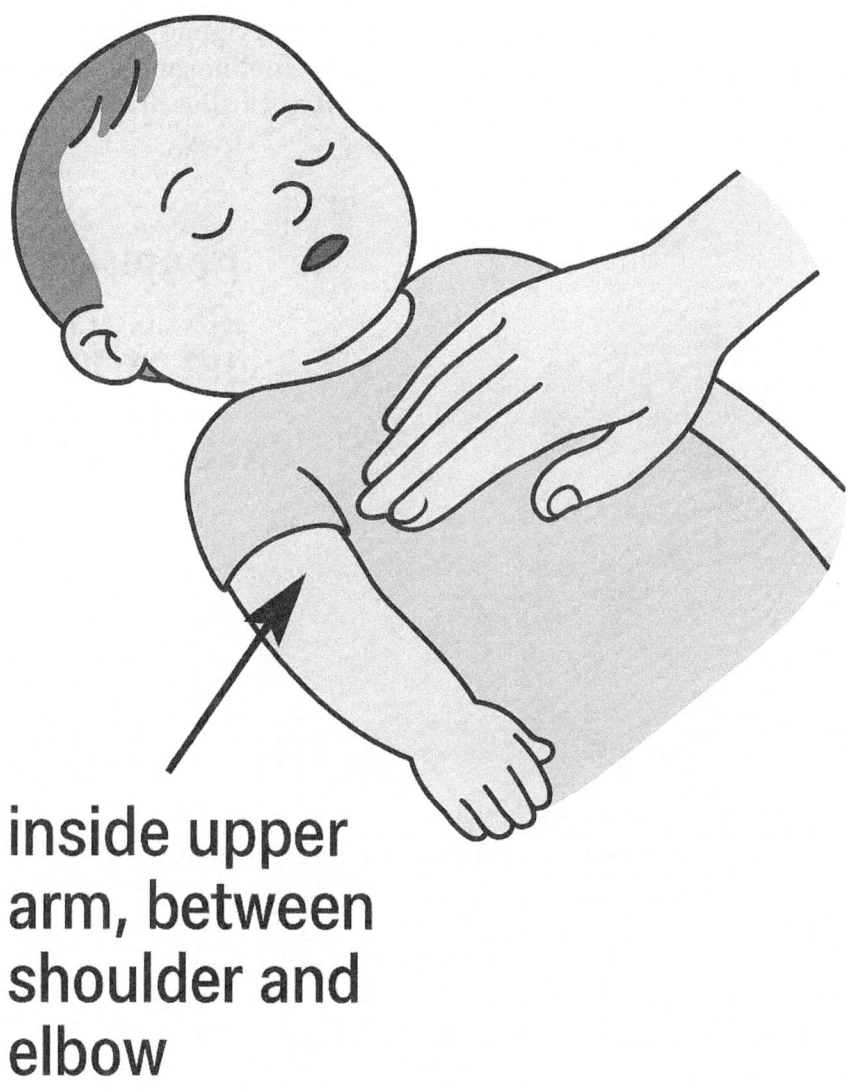

inside upper arm, between shoulder and elbow

Figure 7- Brachial pulse image

It's far more dangerous to hesitate than to act. You cannot make things worse by trying — but you can lose a life by doing nothing.

Many people freeze out of fear of "doing it wrong." You don't have to be confident; you just need courage. Confidence grows from action.

Recognizing "Not Breathing Normally"

Agonal respirations (sporadic gasps, snorting, gurgling) often occur in the first minutes after cardiac arrest. They **are not normal breathing**. If a person is unresponsive and gasping, **treat it as cardiac arrest** and **start compressions**.

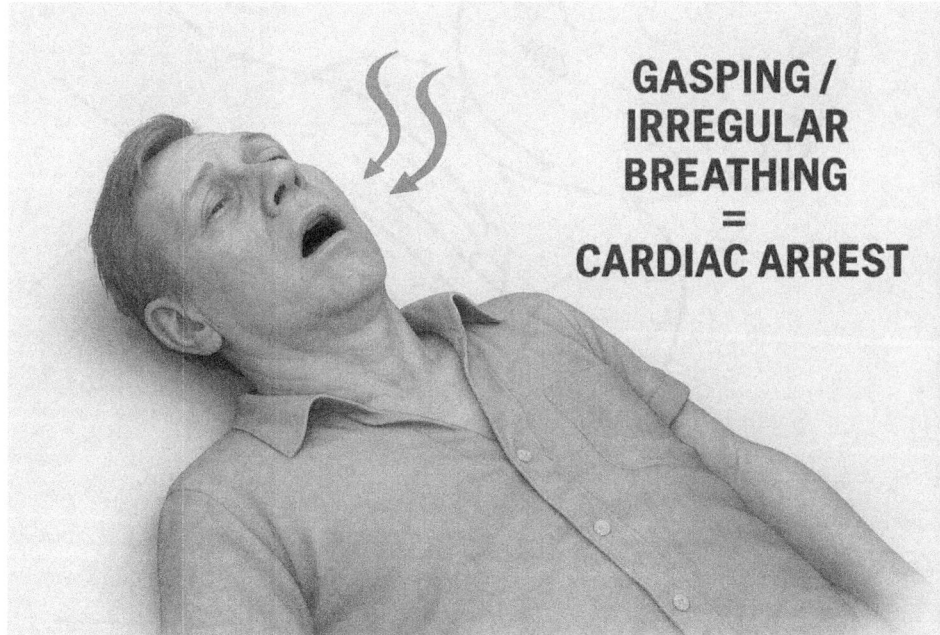

Figure 8- Gasping/ Irregular breathing

1. What It Is

Agonal breathing (or *agonal gasps*) is a reflexive, abnormal pattern of breathing that occurs after the heart has stopped — during the first minutes of cardiac arrest.

It looks like deep, labored, or sporadic gasps, sometimes accompanied by snorting or gurgling sounds.

Even though it appears like breathing, it is not effective respiration — no meaningful oxygen is delivered to the lungs or brain.

2. What Causes It

When cardiac arrest occurs:
- The heart stops pumping blood effectively.
- As a result, oxygen delivery to the brainstem decreases sharply.
- The brainstem's respiratory centers (especially in the medulla oblongata) remain partially active for a short time — they fire sporadic impulses to the muscles that control breathing.
- These impulses cause occasional, reflexive gasps — that's what rescuers see as *agonal breathing*.

So, agonal respirations are a neurological reflex caused by brainstem hypoxia (low oxygen), not true breathing.

3. Why It Matters in CPR
- Agonal breathing is one of the earliest signs of cardiac arrest — often seen in the first 1–3 minutes after the heart stops.
- Lay rescuers and even clinicians sometimes mistake it for real breathing, delaying CPR.
- Recognizing it quickly is critical, because:

Agonal breathing = no pulse, no oxygenation → start Compressions immediately.

When to Start CPR (All Ages)

Start CPR immediately when:
- The person is **unresponsive** and **not breathing** normally (or only gasping).
- There is no **definite pulse** within **10 seconds** (trained rescuers).
- You are **unsure**—when in doubt, **start**.

Courage before confidence: It's safer to start CPR than to hesitate and lose time.

When to Stop CPR

Continue until one of the following occurs:
- **Signs of life/ROSC:** The person breathes normally, moves with purpose, or you feel a definite pulse.
- **AED/EMS takeover:** Trained responders arrive and assume care, or AED advises and guides next steps.
- **You are physically exhausted** and cannot safely continue.
- **The scene becomes unsafe** (fire, traffic, structural danger).
- **A qualified professional** (physician or authorized provider) instructs you to stop.
- **A valid DNR/POLST** is confirmed and clearly applies.

If you **cannot verify** a DNR/POLST **immediately**, treat as **Full Code** and begin/continue resuscitation until clarity is established. If a **DNR** (Do Not Resuscitate) order is visible and confirmed, respect it.

Practical Scene Wisdom

- **Expose the chest when feasible** for accurate hand and **AED pad** placement. If exposure would cause delay, begin over clothing while preparing to expose safely.
- Conduct a **fast hazard scan**: look for needles, medication patches, penetrating objects, pooled fluids, electrical sources, or traffic. Your safety keeps the rescue going.
- If an **AED** arrives, **turn it on immediately** and follow prompts—**resume compressions** right after any shock or analysis.

Micro-Checklist: Start vs. Stop

Start CPR if:
- Unresponsive + not breathing normally (or only gasping)
- No definite pulse within 10 seconds (trained)
- You're unsure

Stop CPR if:
- Normal breathing/pulse returns (ROSC)
- EMS/AED directs and takes over
- You're exhausted or the scene is unsafe

- A qualified professional stops the effort
- A valid DNR/POLST is confirmed and applicable

One line to remember:

If you're wondering whether to start—start. If you're wondering whether to stop—don't, unless one of the clear stop conditions is met.

Chapter 5 – Step-by-Step Guide to CPR

This chapter breaks down what to do for adults, children, and infants. Use it as a practical script you can follow under pressure.

Universal First Steps (All Ages)

1. **Ensure scene safety.**
   Look for traffic, electricity, fluids, weapons, or unstable surfaces.

2. **Check responsiveness.**
   Tap and shout: "Are you OK?" Do not shake (possible spinal injury).

3. **Call for help / Activate EMS.**
   Use speakerphone. Assign tasks specifically: "You in the blue shirt—call 911 and bring the AED."

4. **Check breathing** and—if trained—**check pulse for 5–10 seconds**.
   - **Not breathing normally** (or only gasping) → treat as cardiac arrest.
   - **No definite pulse / unsure** → **start CPR now.**

Priority: Start compressions. Minimize interruptions. Apply the AED the moment it arrives and follow prompts.

Adult CPR (Puberty and up)

Hand Placement & Body Mechanics
- Heel of one hand on the **center of the chest** (lower half of the sternum); other hand on top, fingers interlaced.
- **Elbows locked, shoulders over hands**, straight arms.
- Use a hard, flat surface when possible.

Compression Essentials
- **Rate:** 100–120/min
- **Depth:** at least 2 inches (5 cm) (avoid excessively deep compressions)
- **Recoil:** Allow the chest to fully rise after each compression—no leaning.
- **Interruptions:** Keep to <10 seconds (for breaths, AED rhythm checks, or role switches).

Ventilation (if trained & equipped)
- **Cycle:** 30 compressions: 2 breaths
- **Breaths:** Each over ~1 second, just enough to see visible chest rise (avoid over-ventilating).
- **Airway:** Head-tilt/chin-lift; if trauma suspected, use jaw thrust if trained.
- **Fatigue plan:** Switch compressors every ~2 minutes (about 5 cycles) to maintain depth and rate.

Child CPR (Over 1 year to puberty)

Pulse & Start Criteria
- Use carotid or femoral pulse (trained rescuers). If no definite pulse in ≤10 sec, or unsure, start compressions.
- Technique Adjustments
- Hand(s): One or two hands (based on child size) on the lower half of the sternum.
- Depth: About 2 inches (5 cm) or one-third of the chest's anterior-posterior diameter.
- Rate: 100–120/min with full recoil.
- Ratios
- Single rescuer: 30:2
- Two or more rescuers: 15:2

Tip: If you cannot provide breaths, hands-only CPR is still far better than doing nothing. Add breaths as soon as you are able.

Infant CPR (Birth to 1 year)

Pulse & Start Criteria
- **Check brachial pulse** on the inner upper arm for ≤10 seconds. If absent or uncertain → start CPR.
- **Compression Technique**
- **Single rescuer:** Two-finger technique on the sternum just below the nipple line.
- **Two or more rescuers:** Encircling hands / two-thumb technique (preferred for quality).
- Depth: About 1.5 inches (4 cm) or one-third of chest depth.
- Rate: 100–120/min with full recoil.

Ratios

Single rescuer: 30:2

Two or more rescuers: 15:2 Ventilation Notes Keep the head in a neutral position (avoid overextension).

Deliver gentle breaths over ~1 second each—just until chest rise is seen.

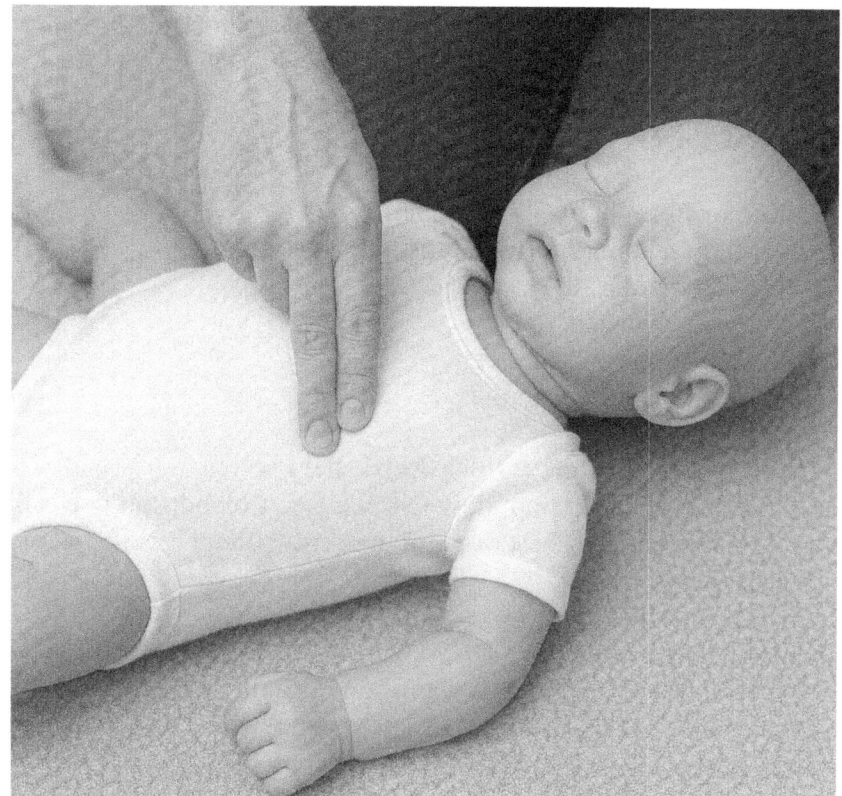

Figures 9 – Infant CPR Two-Finger Technique

Quiz: What's one sign of puberty (besides attitude)?

Growth of underarm or facial hair in boys, breast development in girls.

Putting It Together:

A Step-by-Step Flow (Adults shown; adapt depth/hand use per age)

- **Safety check** → Responsiveness → Call EMS/AED.
- **Breathing & pulse check** (≤10 sec) if trained.
- **Start compressions** in the center of the chest (lower half of sternum).
- Rate 100–120/min, depth ≥2 in (5 cm) for adults, full recoil.

1. **Add breaths** (if trained & barrier available): 30:2
2. Open airway, seal, deliver 1-second breaths with visible chest rise.

- Minimize pauses.
- Resume compressions immediately after breaths and after any AED shock/analysis.

3. **Switch roles** every ~2 minutes to prevent fatigue.

4. **Continue until:**
   - Normal breathing/pulse returns, or
   - AED/EMS takes over, or
   - You are exhausted, or
   - Scene becomes unsafe, or
   - Valid DNR/POLST applies.

Why Chest Recoil Matters (Quick Refresher)
Think of the chest like a pump: down-stroke ejects blood; full rise refills the heart. Leaning on the chest or going too fast without recoil starves the next compression.

Practical Quality Tips
Count out loud or use a metronome app/song beat to hold 100–120/min. Avoid excessive ventilation—over-inflation can reduce blood return to the heart.

Clear commands reduce chaos:
- "Start compressions."
- "You—time us and call out two minutes."
- "AED here—powering on—everyone clear."
- Medication patches & devices: Remove patches (gloved hand) and do not place AED pads over a pacemaker/ICD bulge—offset slightly.

- **Hairy/wet chests:** Improve pad contact (quick dry where pads go; use "wax-strip" trick with spare pads if needed).

Special Notes
- **Opioid overdose**: If available, administer naloxone per local protocol without delaying CPR/AED.

- **Pregnancy**: Perform standard CPR and use an AED as usual; if advanced, a trained team may perform manual uterine displacement—your job is to keep compressions going and apply AED.

- **Trauma:** Prioritize compressions; use jaw-thrust for airway if trained. Control severe bleeding, if possible, without stopping CPR.

One line to remember: Hard, fast, deep, full recoil—minimize pauses, add breaths if trained, power on the AED ASAP.

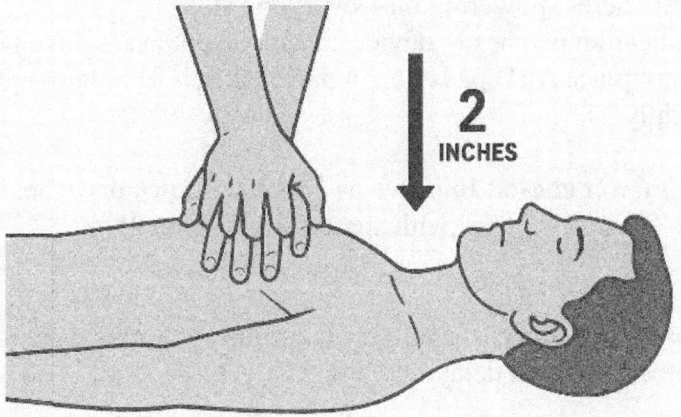

Figures 10 – Correct Hand Position and Chest Recoil Depth

Chapter 6 – AED Basics and How to Use One

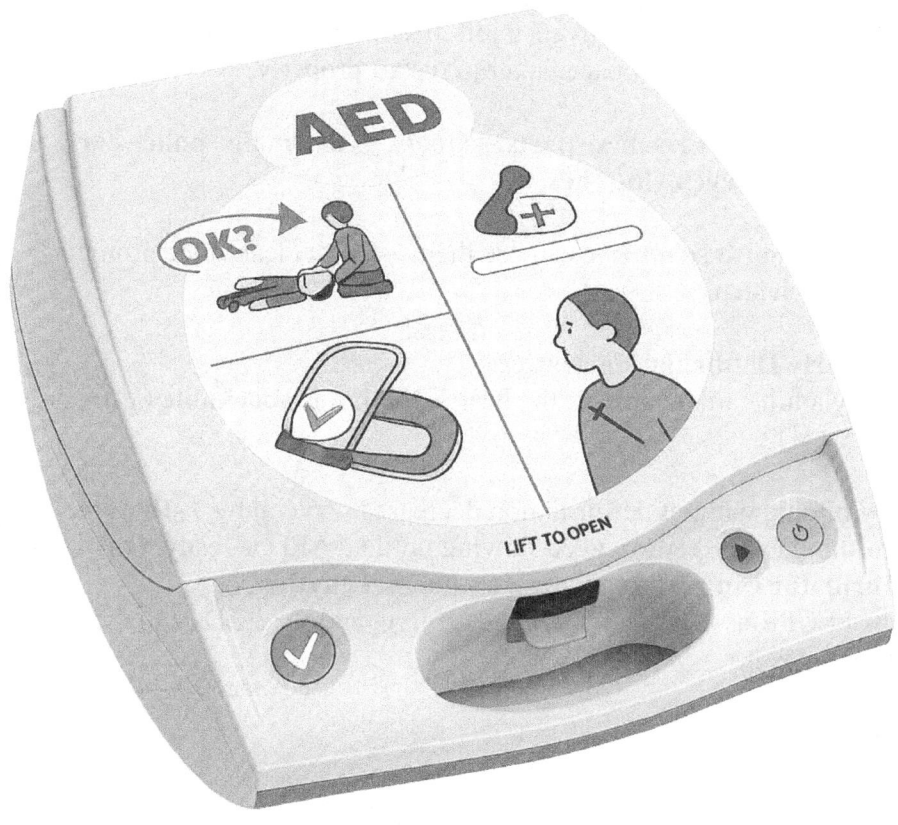

Figure 11- AED

An **Automated External Defibrillator (AED)** analyzes the heart's rhythm and, if necessary, delivers a controlled electrical shock to restore a normal rhythm.

Don't be intimidated by the name — an AED is simply the *external* version of a pacemaker. A pacemaker keeps a heart beating from inside the body; an AED performs the same task from the outside.

If someone with a pacemaker goes into cardiac arrest, it means the device has failed — so it's safe to use an AED on them.

The word *defibrillator* comes from *"de-"* (to reverse) and *"fibrillate"* (to quiver or spasm).

During **ventricular fibrillation (V-fib)** the heart shakes instead of pumping. Defibrillation delivers a jolt to stop the chaotic rhythm and allow the heart's natural pacemaker to restart properly.

You'll now find AEDs in **airports, schools, gyms, malls, police cars, airplanes, and even churches.**

They're designed so *anyone* can use them — with clear voice prompts guiding each step.

Why Early Defibrillation Matters
In many adult cardiac arrests, the heart's rhythm is **shockable** (V-fib or pulseless VT).

Every minute without defibrillation decreases survival by **7–10 percent**. Performing CPR keeps oxygen flowing until an AED is ready. **Only a defibrillator can restart the heart's normal rhythm.**
Think of CPR as keeping the *engine turning*, and the AED as the *spark* that reignites it.

Steps to Use an AED

Turn On the Device
Press the power button and listen. It will speak to you.

Expose the Chest
Cut or remove clothing so the pads stick directly to skin.
If the chest is wet, quickly dry only the areas where pads will go — no need to dry the entire body.

Attach the Pads as Illustrated
- One on the **upper right chest**.
- One on the **lower left side**, below the armpit.
- (Always remember the rule → *High Right / Low Left.*)

Allow the AED to Analyze Rhythm
Step back; make sure no one is touching the victim.

If Advised, Deliver Shock
The device will say, "Shock advised. Press the orange button now."
Announce clearly:

"Everyone clear!" — then press Shock.

Resume CPR Immediately
Right after the shock, perform 2 minutes of CPR (about 5 cycles of 30:2).
The AED will re-analyze automatically and tell you what to do next.

Special Situations
- **Drowning Victim:** Dry only the chest area for pad adhesion.
- **Medication Patch:** Remove it with a gloved hand and wipe the skin clean.
- **Pacemaker Bulge:** Do not place pads directly over the device; offset them slightly.
- **Hairy Chest:** If pads won't stick, use the extra set as a "wax strip." Stick and rip to remove hair, then apply the second set. If the person yells "Ouch!" — they're back! Goal achieved.
- **Infants:** Use infant pads when available. If only adult pads exist, place one in front of the chest and one on the back, sandwiching the heart.

Pregnancy and AED Use
Should you perform CPR or use an AED on a pregnant woman?

Absolutely yes.
When the mother's heart stops, so does the baby's oxygen supply.
By restoring the mother's circulation, you give both a chance to survive.
Even if the mother cannot be saved, maintaining circulation keeps the baby viable until delivery or C-section at the hospital.

Remember: One life in your hands often means two hearts at stake.

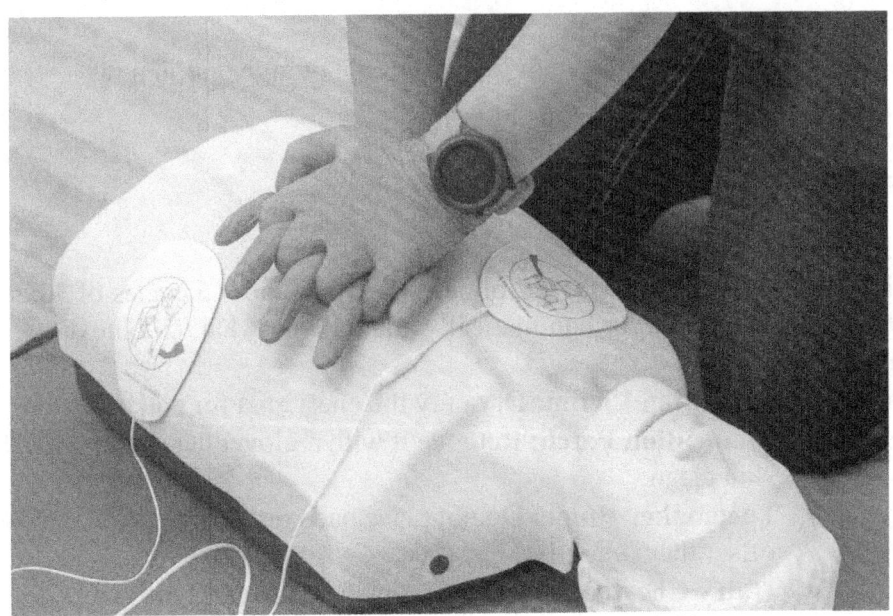

Figure 12 – AED Pad Placement (Adult)

Chapter 7 – Understanding Code Status (Full Code vs DNR)

In healthcare facilities, the term **"Code Status"** determines what life-saving measures will be performed if a patient's heart stops or breathing ceases. Understanding this distinction helps both professionals and families make informed, compassionate choices.

1. Full Code- Do Everything Possible

A **Full Code** means every possible intervention will be attempted — CPR, defibrillation, intubation, and advanced medications. It represents *doing everything medically possible* to restore life.

2. DNR – Do Not Resuscitate

A **DNR order** (Do Not Resuscitate) means the person has chosen *not* to receive CPR or advanced resuscitation efforts if their heart stops.

It is a personal and legal decision — often made to avoid unnecessary suffering or medical futility in terminal conditions.

Reasons patients choose DNR may include:
- Terminal or end-stage illness
- Irreversible brain injury or severe dementia
- Frailty where CPR would cause trauma without restoring function
- A wish to die naturally without aggressive intervention

Respect is key.

A DNR does *not* mean "Do Not Treat." Comfort care, pain relief, and dignity always continue.

3. POLST – Physician Orders for Life-Sustaining Treatment

A **POLST** (or MOLST in some states) expands on the DNR form. It is a **medical order**, signed by a clinician, that specifies exactly which treatments are desired or declined.

Typical sections include:
- Attempt CPR or DNR
- Hospital transfer vs comfort care only
- Antibiotics preferences
- Feeding tubes or IV fluids

Unlike an advance directive, a **POLST follows the patient across settings**—hospital, nursing home, ambulance, or home care—and must be honored by all licensed providers.

If code status is **unknown, always treat the patient as Full Code** until official documents are reviewed or family/legal representatives confirm otherwise. "When in doubt, act to save — clarity can come later." A delay while searching for papers can cost a life; documentation can be reviewed afterward.

Balancing Ethics and Emotion
- Sometimes emotion and ethics collide:
- A young responder wants to help, but legal orders forbid it.
- A nurse feels guilt for following a DNR that ends in death.
- These moments test not only policy but the heart.
- The ethical standard is **autonomy and dignity** — the right of each person to choose.
- The emotional standard is **compassion** — acting with kindness even when the choice is to let go.

Good care isn't only about doing more; it's about doing what's right.

Real-World Example

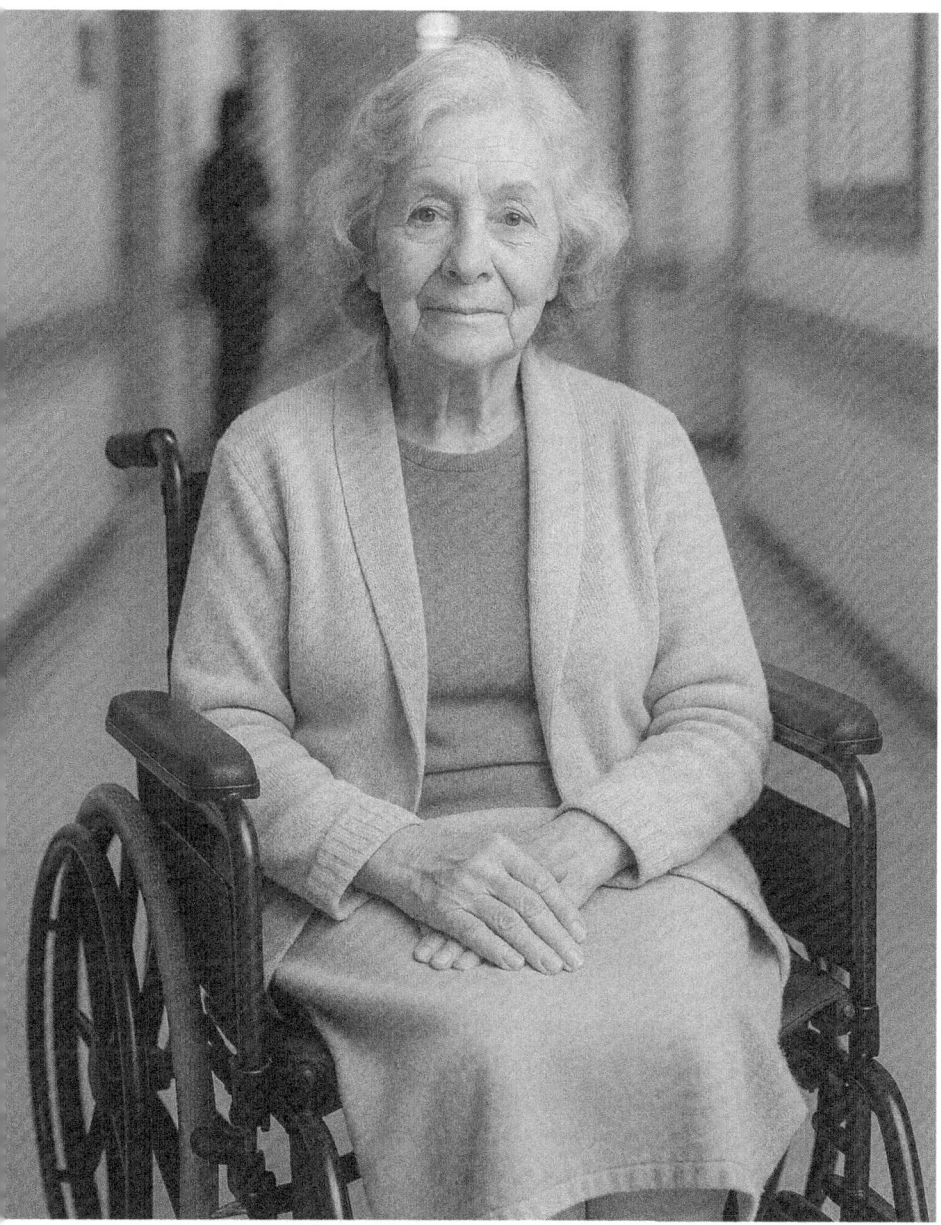

Figure 13- Mrs. Pam sits quietly in the hallway
The Mrs. Pam Case – A Second Chance

At a long-term care facility, Mrs. Pam a newly admitted patient. As she sat quietly in the hallway, unaware that within minutes her heartbeat will become the focus of every pair of hands on the unit went into cardiac arrest. This happened before staff could confirm her chart or code status.

Following California protocol, she was treated as **Full Code** and CPR began instantly.

Paramedics arrived and transferred her to the hospital while still unconscious. Two weeks later, she returned — sitting upright in a wheelchair.

One of the nurses who had performed CPR walked toward her smiling, saying: "Mrs. Pam, I'm so happy to see you! I was one of the nurses who did CPR on you." Mrs. Pam looked at her, frowned, and said:

"You're the one who brought me back? Why did you bring me back?" That moment stayed with all of us.

It was a reminder that CPR is not just a medical act — but an encounter with destiny, where faith, choice, and physiology intersect.

Behind every compression is a heartbeat shared, and behind every rescue is a story that changes both lives — the rescuer and the rescued.

Scenario – The Power of Early Action
In another incident at the prison, an inmate overdosed and went into cardiac arrest. After CPR and transfer to the hospital, he survived. When he returned, he was holding a bible in his hand, thanking God and asking everyone to repent. Moments like these stay with you forever.

The Prison Inmate's Story
Again, at this **Level 4 maximum-security prison** where I worked as a nurse. While performing routine duties on the yard (secured outdoor where inmates engage in sporting activities), we observed an inmate appeared to be in medical distress. **The emergency alarm was activated** immediately, in accordance with prison protocol. **Responding correctional officers announced "Man Down"** over the radio and secured the area for medical response. We initiated assessment and appropriate medical intervention.

We rushed him into the clinic just before he became unresponsive. I grabbed scissors and cut open his shirt to start compressions.

Paramedics arrived minutes later and transferred him to the hospital.

Days afterward, he returned — alive, alert, and agitated. As soon as he saw me, he shouted across the room, "Gumbo! Why did you cut my shirt? You owe me a new one!"

We all laughed — but inside, I felt deep gratitude.
The shirt could be replaced; his heartbeat could not.

Lessons These Moments Teach

Time is everything.
Each story reinforces that every second matters more than perfection. Acting immediately — even imperfectly — buys life.

Courage beats fear.
Everyone hesitates at first. Training gives confidence, but courage begins before confidence arrives.

Teamwork saves lives.
A clear voice, quick assignments, and mutual trust turn chaos into choreography.

Humor heals after the crisis.
Laughter after survival isn't disrespect — it's relief. It's proof that life has returned.

Every rescue changes you.
After each event, you carry the memory — sometimes heavy, sometimes joyful — but always sacred.

Reflection
CPR isn't only about compressions and breaths; it's about **connection**. When you kneel beside a person whose heart has stopped, you're holding a moment suspended between life and loss. After they've lost their heartbeat, you're not only lending your hands- you're sharing your heart.

Whether in a hospital hallway or a prison cell, that moment demands everything you have — knowledge, courage, and compassion. Sometimes the story ends in laughter, sometimes in tears, but always in meaning.

Every act of resuscitation is an act of hope.
Even when the outcome is uncertain, the effort itself is a victory — proof that humanity still answers the call to help.

Chapter 8 – Common Mistakes and Myths About CPR

Even the most well-meaning rescuers hesitate — not because they don't care, but because they have been told myths that cause doubt or fear. Let's correct the most common ones so you can act without hesitation when it truly counts.

Myth #1: "I might hurt the person."

Reality:
Yes, ribs might crack. That's normal. Broken ribs can heal — a stopped heart cannot. The goal is circulation, not comfort.
In training, we say, *"If you hear a crack, that means you're doing it right."*
It means compressions are deep enough to move the heart and pump blood to the brain.

Myth #2: "I can't perform CPR because I'm not certified."

Reality:
Certification helps refine your technique, but it's **not required** to save a life.

If someone collapses and you start hands-only compressions, you are protected by the **Good Samaritan Law** in most countries, including the United States.

The law shields rescuers from liability when they act in good faith to help someone in an emergency.

Myth #3: "Mouth-to-mouth is always required."

Reality:
The American Heart Association now recommends **hands-only CPR** for adults if you're untrained or uncomfortable with rescue breaths.

Just push hard and fast in the center of the chest — that alone doubles or triples the chance of survival.

If you have a **barrier device** (like a pocket mask) or are trained, adding 2 breaths after every 30 compressions is ideal.

Myth #4: "If they're gasping, they're breathing."

Reality:
When the heart stops, the brain may trigger reflex gasps known as **agonal respirations** — irregular, shallow, or snorting breaths.

These are **not true breathing.**
If someone is unresponsive and gasping without normal breathing, start CPR immediately.

Myth #5: "CPR doesn't work outside hospitals."

Reality:
Thousands of people survive cardiac arrest every year because a bystander — an ordinary person like you — refused to stand by. Survival often depends on what happens before paramedics arrive. CPR buys time, keeping the brain and organs alive until professional help can restart the heart with a defibrillator.

Myth #6: "I might be sued if I perform CPR."

Reality:
Good Samaritan Laws protect you as long as your actions are reasonable and in good faith. In fact, failure to act when you could have helped can lead to regret that lasts much longer than any fear of legal risk.
Act with compassion, follow basic principles, and you've done the right thing.

Myth #7: "It's too late."

Reality:
Even if a person looks pale or lifeless, CPR can still make a difference. Many people have been revived after several minutes without a pulse.

Until rigor mortis sets in or a medical professional declares death, **it's never too late to try.**

Myth #8: "You need special equipment."

Reality:
All you need is your hands and a willing heart.
CPR can be done anywhere — at home, on the roadside, in a store, or at the gym.
Every minute counts. The average ambulance response time in the U.S. is 4–8 minutes — and the brain begins to die after 4.

Myth #9: "I'll freeze under pressure."

Reality:
You might — and that's okay. Everyone feels fear the first time.
But courage doesn't mean you don't feel fear — it means you act anyway.
Remember the motto of this book:

"You don't need confidence to save a life — only courage. Confidence comes later."

Final Thought for This Chapter
- There's no perfect rescuer.
- There's only a willing one.

A shaky, uncertain rescuer who acts will always save more lives than a confident bystander who hesitates. You don't need a degree to restart a heartbeat — just the will to try. Hands save hearts, Courage saves lives.

Chapter 9 – Emotional and Ethical Aspects of Resuscitation

Performing CPR is not just a technical skill — it's an emotional experience. Each rescue carries a mix of adrenaline, hope, fear, and humanity. Whether you're a nurse, caregiver, or bystander, the moment you kneel beside a lifeless body and start compressions, you become part of that person's story.

The Emotional Reality
CPR can be intense, both physically and mentally. Even trained professionals experience moments of doubt afterward:

- Did I do it right?
- Was it enough?
- What if they don't make it?

These questions are normal. They show compassion.
But remember this: **Doing something is always better than doing nothing.**

Even if the outcome isn't what you hoped for, your effort mattered. Your actions gave someone a fighting chance they would not have had otherwise.

For Healthcare Workers
In hospitals, nursing homes, or prisons, healthcare staff often face "code blues".

The constant exposure to death and emergency can lead to emotional fatigue.

You might feel numb after repeated losses or replay failed resuscitations in your mind. This is called **Code Fatigue** or **Rescuer Burnout.**
The key is to **debrief, talk, and heal.**

After a code event, gather your team, share thoughts, and allow emotions to surface. Many institutions conduct "post-code debriefs" not only to review performance but also to process the emotional toll.

Remember: "You can't pour from an empty cup. Heal the healer, and the care continues."

The COVID Experience

During the COVID-19 pandemic, I worked at a correctional facility where nearly every day someone went into cardiac arrest. We performed CPR countless times — often wearing layers of PPE, sweating, and fearing exposure ourselves.

There were days when exhaustion felt heavier than the patient on the gurney.

Yet, we kept going, because even one success — one heartbeat returning — made it all worth it.

That season taught me that **CPR is both a science and an act of faith.** Each compression is a prayer for life.

For Families

Watching CPR performed on a loved one is one of the hardest moments a family can experience. Some cry and pray; others stand frozen; a few beg the rescuers to stop.

- When the person survives, gratitude floods the room.
- When they don't, families often ask, *"Did we do the right thing?"*
- The answer is yes — because the decision came from love.
- Whether the outcome was life or loss, compassion was the motive.

Debrief Example

After one difficult case during COVID, I remember sitting with two RNs who had tears in their eyes. One said,

"I feel like we fail every time they don't come back."
I replied,

"We never fail when we try. Failure is standing by and doing nothing."

That became our mantra for months.

Trying means caring, and caring is what makes us human.

Final Message of This Chapter
CPR is more than compressions and breaths. It's empathy in action — a universal gesture of love that crosses race, culture, religion, and language.

When your hands press down on another human's chest, you are saying:

"Your life matters enough for me to fight for it."
Never underestimate the emotional courage it takes to be that person.

Chapter 10 – Choking (Adults, Infants, Pregnant & LifeVac)

Choking is another life-threatening emergency where **seconds truly count.** When the airway becomes blocked, oxygen cannot reach the lungs or the brain. Within minutes, the person can lose consciousness, and cardiac arrest soon follows. Recognizing and responding quickly can mean the difference between life and death.

Recognizing Choking
- Inability to speak or breathe
- Hands clutching the throat (the universal choking sign)
- High-pitched wheezing or no sound at all
- Bluish lips or fingernails
- Panicked expression or grasping for air

If someone can cough or talk, encourage them to keep coughing. If they can't make a sound — **they need your help immediately.**

Adult Choking Procedure
Ask firmly, "Are you choking?" If they nod or cannot speak, act at once. Stand behind the person and wrap your arms around their waist. Make a fist and place the thumb side above the navel (but below the sternum).

Grasp the fist with your other hand and perform **quick, inward-and-upward thrusts.** Use a motion as if you are trying to lift them off their feet. **Alternate 5 back blows and 5 abdominal thrusts.**

Repeat until the object is expelled or they become unresponsive. If they lose consciousness, **gently lower them to the ground and begin CPR.** Before each breath, quickly look into the mouth — if you see an object and can easily remove it with two fingers, do so. Never perform blind finger sweeps.

Remember: Abdominal thrusts generate air pressure from the lungs to dislodge an object — similar to a small cough from the inside out.

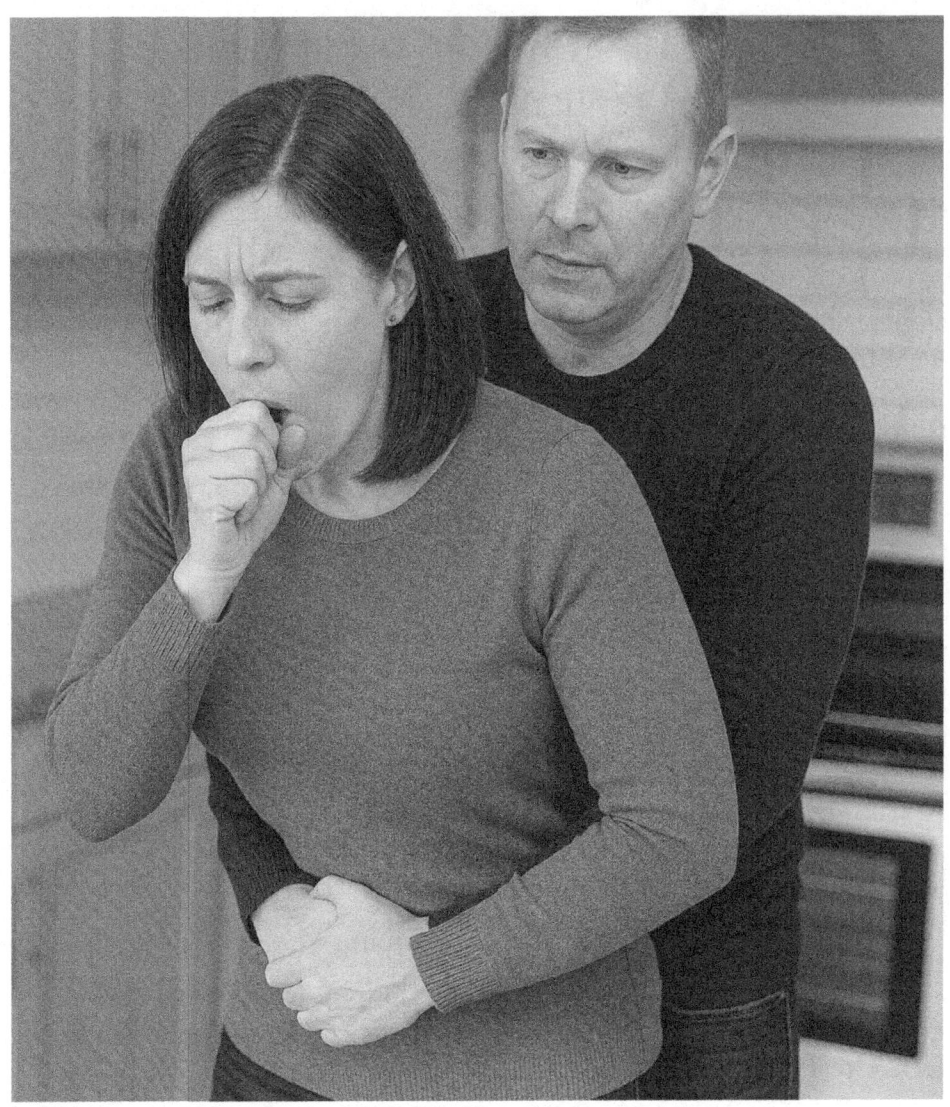

Figure 14- Adult Choking Abdominal thrusts

Pregnant or Obese Victims

For pregnant individuals or obese victims where abdominal thrusts are difficult or unsafe:

- Perform **chest thrusts** instead of abdominal thrusts.
- Place your hands at the center of the chest, the same location used for CPR compressions.
- Deliver sharp, inward thrusts until the object is expelled or the person collapses.

For pregnant patients, this reduces pressure on the abdomen and protects the baby while still creating the needed force to clear the airway.

Infant Choking (Under 1 Year)

Infants are especially vulnerable because their airways are small, and they explore objects with their mouths.

Support the baby's head and neck firmly. Lay the infant face-down along your forearm, with the head slightly lower than the body. Deliver **5 firm back slaps** between the shoulder blades using the heel of your hand.

If the object does not dislodge, **turn the infant face-up** and perform **5 gentle chest thrusts** with two fingers just below the nipple line.

Alternate 5 back slaps and 5 chest thrusts until the airway is clear or the infant becomes unresponsive.

If unresponsive, start infant CPR immediately and call for help.

Tip: Never perform abdominal thrusts on infants — their organs are too delicate and unprotected.

LifeVac and New Airway Devices

In recent years, devices like **LifeVac**, DeChoker, and similar portable suction tools have become popular in homes, schools, restaurants, and care facilities.

These devices use one-way valves to create suction that removes an airway obstruction in seconds when traditional methods fail. They are non-invasive, require no training, and can be used on adults and children.

Important: Always call 911 even if the object is removed. Choking victims should be checked by medical professionals for throat injury or secondary complications.

Preventing Choking

- Cut food into small pieces for children and elderly individuals.
- Avoid talking or laughing while eating.
- Keep small objects, coins, and toys away from infants.
- Educate caregivers and teachers about first aid responses.
- Prevention is the best cure — awareness saves lives long before emergencies happen.

Reflection

Choking emergencies remind us that life is fragile and fleeting — sometimes hanging on a single breath.
When someone can't breathe, your quick action becomes their lifeline. Every back blow, every thrust, every second of calm focus says one thing louder than panic ever could:

"I will fight for your next breath."

Hands, courage, and compassion — once again, the same formula that saves hearts — also saves airways.

Hands save hearts.

Courage saves lives.

Chapter 11– Living Through CPR: Realities, Gratitude & Courage

Every CPR attempt carries a story — a collision of science, faith, fear, and courage.

Sometimes the outcome is miraculous. Other times it's humbling. But in every case, it's deeply human- because when you perform CPR, you're standing at the intersection of this life and eternity.

The Realities
When someone's heart stops, you have just **four minutes** before significant brain damage begins.

Those four minutes decide everything — life, death, or lifelong disability. Performing CPR is exhausting. It's physical work — pushing hard and fast on the chest, counting compressions, giving breaths, following commands, waiting for help.

And yet, amid the chaos, something profound happens:

You become the difference between hope and despair.
Even if paramedics take over later, those first moments are yours — the ones that truly matter. Those hands, your hands- make the greatest difference. You may not be a doctor, but in that moment, you are someone's only chance.

Gratitude

There's an incredible moment that happens sometimes after successful CPR.

The person you helped — once pale and lifeless — might one day look at you, breathing and alive.

Maybe they thank you. Maybe they don't remember you. But you'll remember.

- You'll remember the sound of their first gasp.
- You'll remember the sigh of relief from others watching.
- You'll remember that your courage gave someone another sunrise.

Like the inmate who had overdosed and returned from the hospital holding a Bible.

He later approached us in the clinic and said,
"Thank you for saving my life. God sent you for me. I'm going to change my life." That moment reminded me why I do what I do. Not for recognition — but for redemption.

The Humor That Heals
Not every story ends in tears — some end in laughter. Like the inmate who yelled, "You owe me a new shirt!" after I cut his uniform open to start CPR. Or the patient who said,

"Why did you bring me back? I was resting!"
Even in those moments, there's healing.

Because it means CPR worked — life returned, breath resumed, and the heart found its rhythm again.

Courage Before Confidence
In every CPR class I teach, I tell my students:

"You don't have to be confident to save a life — you just need courage. Because courage comes before confidence."

Courage acts while confidence grows from action.
That trembling first step — kneeling beside a collapsed person and pressing your hands on their chest — is what builds confidence later. You can't practice bravery in theory; you prove it in action.

Even if your hands shake, **shaking hands can still restart a heart.**

When Things Don't Go as Hoped
There are times when CPR doesn't succeed — and those moments can weigh heavily. You may feel like you failed. But let this truth stay with you:

Failure is not defined by outcome, but by inaction.
You showed up. You tried. You gave someone a chance.
That alone places you among the courageous few who choose action over fear.

What CPR Teaches Us About Life
- CPR teaches more than a medical skill — it teaches **resilience**.
- Every compression symbolizes persistence.
- Every breath symbolizes hope.
- Every AED shock symbolizes second chances.
- It reminds us that in life, just like in resuscitation, every small effort matters.

Each heartbeat restored begins with someone who refused to give up. In resuscitation, as in life, every effort counts- and every heartbeat matters.

Final Thought

When you step forward to perform CPR, you are joining the universal rhythm of humanity — a rhythm that says, *"Life is sacred, and I will fight for it."*

- Even when no one's watching.
- Even when you're afraid.
- Even when your hands tremble.
- Because compassion beats stronger than fear.

Because compassion beats stronger than fear.

Hands save hearts.
Courage saves lives.

<u>Courage before confidence — always.</u>

Conclusion – The Power to Save a Life

CPR is more than a medical procedure — it's a universal language of hope. Every time a person learns, teaches, or performs CPR, the world becomes a little safer. The moment you decide to act, you bridge the gap between life and loss.

- You don't have to be perfect.
- You don't have to be fearless.
- You just have to **care enough to start.**
- Every compression you perform is a heartbeat shared.
- Every breath given is a whisper of hope.
- Every act of courage echoes louder than fear.

If you ever doubt your ability, remember: When someone's heart stops, they need *your hands, your will, your presence.* Not your perfection.
The power to save a life is not reserved for heroes — it belongs to anyone with compassion and courage. You don't need a title, uniform, or certification to make that difference. You simply need to care enough to try. That's not just CPR, that's Compassion in motion.

<u>Courage before confidence — always.</u>

About the Author

Munashe Davies Gumbo is a Nurse, BLS/CPR Instructor (AHA, Red Cross, HSI), and the Founder of **OM Good Samaritan** — a healthcare staffing and education organization serving California's Bay Area, Central Coast, and Central Valley.

With over a decade of clinical and educational experience, Munashe has taught countless caregivers, nurses, and community members to respond confidently in emergencies. He blends technical training with storytelling to make lifesaving knowledge approachable, memorable, and empowering.

Through his *Life & Recovery Series*, he seeks to bridge the gap between clinical knowledge and human compassion — teaching not just *how* to save a life, but *why it matters*.

"You don't need confidence to begin. You need courage — because courage comes first, and confidence follows."

For more resources and training programs, visit:
www.goodsamaritanca.com   books@goodsamaritanca.com

Back Cover Summary

When a heart stops, seconds matter.
CPR Made Simple turns fear into action and complexity into confidence. Written in everyday language by nurse and instructor **Munashe Gumbo**, this book transforms CPR from a technical skill into a compassionate act — teaching you how to:

- Perform effective CPR (adult, child, and infant)
- Use an AED with confidence
- Respond to choking emergencies (including pregnant victims and infants)
- Understand Full Code vs. DNR status
- Overcome fear, hesitation, and emotional barriers

With real-life examples — from nursing homes to correctional facilities — this guide brings CPR to life with warmth, clarity, and purpose. You'll finish this book not only knowing *how* to save a life but *believing you can*. Because courage comes before confidence. And every heartbeat restored begins with that first moment of courage.

I wrote this book to help you move — to give you the confidence, clarity, and compassion to act when someone's heartbeat stops.
Because in that moment, your hands may be the only hands that matter. You're not just reviving a body — you're defending a story, a family, and a future.

END OF BOOK

© 2025 Munashe Davies Gumbo. All Rights

Life & Recovery Series—Book 1

Publisher: OM Good Samaritan

books@goodsamaritanca.com

www.goodsamaritanca.com

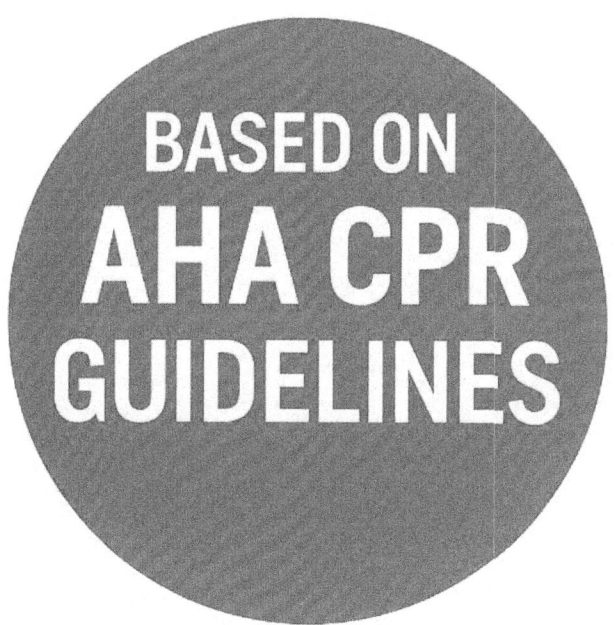

Made in the USA
Coppell, TX
19 January 2026

68040987R00036